The Mystery Of Ehlers-Danlos Syndrome

Living life to the fullest with hypermobility eds and vascular eds, navigating the complex world of ehlers-danlos syndrome

Minnie H. Lewis

Introduction

Have you ever felt like your body was made of paper and glue, coming apart at the slightest touch? Imagine living a life where every stretch, every step, every twist could result in pain or injury.

This is not just a fantasy for thousands of people throughout the world; it is a daily reality.

Welcome to the mysterious world of Ehlers-Danlos Syndrome.

We will dig deeply into the complexities of Ehlers-Danlos Syndrome (EDS) on this captivating adventure. We will investigate its riddle, its far-reaching impact on people impacted, and the never-ending quest for knowledge and remedies. This book shines a light on the complicated network of EDS, with the primary goal of offering information and empowerment to people who face its problems.

The Significance of the book

It is critical to recognize that EDS is more than just a medical illness; it is a life-changing event that impacts people in a variety of ways. This book offers a doorway to information whether you are a medical professional looking to improve your understanding, a patient looking for affirmation and direction, or a family member looking to help a loved one. It strives to provide you with the knowledge, skills, and insights you need to efficiently navigate the particular maze of EDS.

We will answer your concerns, give important advice on living with EDS, and investigate the most recent research and improvements on these pages. We are here to light the way forward, to provide hope and resilience in the midst of a difficult road.

Prepare to embark on a life-changing trip as we explore the world of Ehlers-Danlos Syndrome, unraveling its secrets and discovering the power that exists inside people who live with it.

What exactly is Ehlers-Danlos Syndrome

Ehlers-Danlos syndrome (EDS) is a collection of genetic connective tissue illnesses that predominantly affect your skin, joints, and blood vessel walls. Connective tissue is a complex collection of proteins and other substances that provide your body's underlying structures strength and suppleness.

EDS is defined as a deficiency in the synthesis or structure of collagen, a protein that is essential in these connective tissues.

The primary features of EDS include:

1. **Joint Hypermobility:** People with EDS frequently have hypermobile (extra flexible) joints, which can contribute to dislocations, joint discomfort, and instability.

2. **Skin Abnormalities:** EDS can cause hyperelastic, delicate skin that is easily bruised, scarred, and torn.

3. **Vascular difficulties:** Some EDS subtypes might have serious vascular difficulties, including the

danger of artery or organ rupture, which can be fatal.

4. **Internal Organs Involvement:** EDS can impact internal organs such as the heart, lungs, and gastrointestinal tract, resulting in a variety of difficulties.

EDS is a complicated illness with several subtypes, each with unique features and hereditary reasons. Some subtypes are minor, while others can be severe, offering substantial obstacles to people who are affected. Individuals' intensity and particular symptoms might vary greatly.

EDS diagnosis and management often necessitate a multidisciplinary approach including healthcare experts from many disciplines, such as geneticists, orthopedic specialists, dermatologists, and physical therapists, because of the vast spectrum of symptoms and associated problems. Physical therapy, pain management, and, in certain situations, surgical procedures are used to treat and manage specific symptoms.

It is crucial to highlight that EDS is a lifelong illness, and people with EDS frequently need to make changes to their lifestyle and healthcare routines to improve their well-being and quality of life. Early diagnosis and an intelligent approach to managing EDS can make a big impact on the lives of individuals affected.

What causes EDS

Mutations in genes that influence the synthesis or structure of collagen or elastin, two of the primary proteins in connective tissue, cause Ehlers-Danlos syndrome (EDS). Connective tissue is a complex collection of proteins and other substances that provide your body's underlying structures strength and suppleness.

EDS may be inherited in several ways. Some kinds of EDS are autosomal dominant, which implies that only one copy of the defective gene from one parent is required to create the disorder. Other varieties of EDS are inherited in an autosomal recessive fashion, which implies that the disorder requires two copies of the defective gene, one from each parent. Other kinds of EDS are produced by new mutations in the individual's genes.

Depending on the kind of EDS, the precise gene mutation that causes it differs. The mutation is known in some cases, but not in others.

Genetic mutations that can cause different types of EDS:

- Mutations in genes that code for collagen types I, III, or V produce hypermobile EDS (hEDS).

- Mutations in genes that code for collagen type I produce classical EDS (cEDS).

- Vascular EDS (vEDS) is caused by mutations in the collagen type III gene.

- Kyphoscoliotic EDS (kEDS) is caused by mutations in the collagen type VI gene.

It is crucial to remember that not everyone with EDS has a family history of the disorder. New mutations can develop in anybody at any time.

If you have EDS, you should consult your doctor regarding the possibility of passing the condition on to your children. Your doctor can also assist you in understanding the hereditary risks of EDS and making educated family planning decisions.

How common is EDS, and who is affected

Ehlers-Danlos Syndrome (EDS) is considered an uncommon disorder, however, determining its actual incidence can be difficult due to underdiagnosis and the vast range of EDS types and symptoms. The prevalence of EDS varies depending on the subtype. Here's an outline of its prevalence and typical victims:

1. **Prevalence:** The total prevalence of EDS is believed to be 1 in 5,000 people. However, depending on the kind of EDS, this figure may vary greatly. The hypermobility kind of EDS, for example, is the most frequent and may be more widespread, but the vascular type is uncommon.

2. **Gender and Age:** EDS can affect people of any age, gender, or ethnicity. Because it is a hereditary disorder, it might be present from birth. EDS is usually identified in childhood or early adulthood as symptoms grow more

severe, however, some people may not be diagnosed until later in life.

3. **Familial Occurrence:** EDS is a genetic illness that can be passed down through families. If a parent has EDS, their children may inherit the disorder, albeit the particular subtype and severity may differ between generations.

4. **Hereditary Connective Tissue Disorders:** EDS is one of several hereditary connective tissue illnesses. These disorders impact the body's connective tissues, resulting in symptoms such as joint hypermobility, skin fragility, and vascular problems. Other connective tissue illnesses, such as Marfan syndrome, may exhibit certain clinical characteristics similar to EDS.

5. **Underdiagnosis:** EDS is frequently misdiagnosed or underdiagnosed, owing to the fact that its symptoms might be vague or overlap with other disorders. Many people with EDS may experience delayed diagnosis and treatment as a result of this.

It is critical to recognize that EDS is a complicated and multidimensional disorder. EDS patients can have a wide range of symptoms and severity levels, ranging from moderate to severe. A timely and correct diagnosis is critical for properly treating the illness and enhancing the quality of life for persons afflicted with EDS.

The different types of EDS, and how they vary

Ehlers-Danlos Syndrome (EDS) is a collection of inherited connective tissue illnesses that are distinguished by distinct genetic abnormalities and clinical symptoms. Here's a rundown of the main forms of EDS and how they differ:

1. Hypermobility EDS (hEDS):

- This is the most frequent kind of EDS.
- It is largely distinguished by joint hypermobility, which refers to the ability of joints to move beyond their usual range of motion.
- People with hEDS may feel joint discomfort, easy bruising, and soft, velvety skin.
- It is not characterized by the significant skin and blood vessel signs found in other EDS types.

2. Classical EDS (cEDS):

- Classical EDS is distinguished by skin hyperextensibility (the ability to stretch the skin more than usual) and joint hypermobility.

- People with cEDS are more likely to develop atrophic, "cigarette paper" scars.

- Common symptoms include easy bruising, joint dislocations, and joint discomfort.

3. Vascular EDS (vEDS):

- Vascular EDS is one of the most severe kinds, with the possibility of life-threatening consequences.

- It is distinguished by fragile blood arteries and internal organs, which raises the risk of arterial and organ rupture.

- Skin involvement is less common in vEDS than in other forms.

4. Kyphoscoliotic EDS (kEDS):

- This kind is distinguished by severe muscular hypotonia at birth, scoliosis, hypermobility of joints, and fragile skin.

- People with kEDS may develop increasing kyphoscoliosis (a form of spine curvature) and muscular weakness.

5. Arthrochalasia EDS (aEDS):

- Arthrochalasia EDS is distinguished by significant joint hypermobility, joint dislocations, and a proclivity for kyphoscoliosis.

- It is also linked to weak and hyperextensible skin.

6. Dermatosparaxis EDS (dEDS):

- dEDS is distinguished by extremely delicate, sagging skin that is prone to ripping and bruising.

- In most cases, joint hypermobility is minor, and additional systemic symptoms are uncommon.

7. **Brittle Cornea Syndrome (BCS)**: Brittle Cornea Syndrome (BCS) is a condition in which the cornea becomes brittle.

- BCS is connected to EDS and is distinguished by a thin, brittle cornea.

- It may also include joint hypermobility and modest skin changes.

8. Musculocontractural EDS (mcEDS):

- Congenital muscular weakness, joint contractures, and specific facial traits define mcEDS.

- There may also be joint hypermobility and cutaneous involvement.

Each kind of EDS has its own set of diagnostic criteria, and a genetic test is usually needed to confirm the subtype. It's crucial to note that symptoms within various categories can overlap significantly, and people with EDS may not cleanly fall into a single group. An accurate diagnosis is required for proper management and therapy.

How EDS diagnosed

Ehlers-Danlos Syndrome (EDS) is diagnosed by a combination of clinical examination, family history review, and, in some cases, genetic testing. Below are outline of the EDS diagnosis process:

1. Clinical Assessment:

- The initial evaluation is usually performed by a healthcare expert, such as a rheumatologist or geneticist.

- The healthcare professional will examine the patient's medical history, and family history, and do a comprehensive physical examination to detect the signs and symptoms of EDS.

2. Family History Assessment:

- EDS is a hereditary disorder that can be passed down through families. A considerable family history of EDS or symptoms connected to the disease may trigger concern.

- Documenting family history is critical for identifying probable inheritance patterns.

3. Beighton Score:

- Joint hypermobility is measured using a Beighton score. It consists of a battery of tests designed to assess the flexibility of various joints in the body. A higher Beighton score indicates more joint hypermobility, which is frequent in several EDS subtypes.

4. The Ghent Criteria:

- The Ghent Criteria are clinical diagnostic criteria for classifying and diagnosing various kinds of EDS.

- These criteria consider factors such as skin involvement, joint hypermobility, and family history.

- Different subtypes of EDS have different diagnostic criteria that must be satisfied.

5. Genetic Analysis:

- Genetic testing may be required in certain individuals to confirm the precise EDS subtype.

- Genetic testing can detect the existence of mutations in EDS-related genes. Mutations in distinct genes have been related to various forms of EDS.

- Genetic testing is especially relevant when the diagnosis is ambiguous or a certain subtype is suspected based on clinical symptoms.

6. Other Tests:

- Additional tests may be requested to examine particular features of EDS depending on the clinical presentation and probable subtype. Skin biopsies, imaging investigations, and heart exams are examples of these examinations.

7. Consulting Experts:

- Because of the vast spectrum of symptoms associated with EDS, patients may need to see a variety of experts, such as dermatologists, orthopedic surgeons, or cardiologists, to examine and treat particular difficulties.

It is crucial to highlight that EDS is a complicated and varied syndrome that can be difficult to diagnose owing to comorbidity with other connective tissue disorders. As a result, a multidisciplinary strategy including several healthcare providers is frequently required to guarantee correct diagnosis and appropriate therapy. A validated EDS diagnosis can also assist in guiding therapy and symptom management measures.

Why are many doctors not informed about EDS

Many doctors and healthcare workers may be under-informed about Ehlers-Danlos Syndrome (EDS) for a variety of reasons, including:

1. **Rare Condition**: EDS is an uncommon disorder, and healthcare practitioners may not come across it regularly in their work. Because of the syndrome's rarity, it may not be a focus of their medical education or training.

2. **Lack of Awareness:** Medical practitioners may be unaware of the existence of EDS. Some clinicians may be unfamiliar with the clinical characteristics, diagnostic criteria, or subgroups of EDS.

3. **Variability and Complexity**: EDS is a complicated and extremely varied condition. It might appear with a variety of symptoms that coincide with other medical disorders, making diagnosis difficult. Symptom variability might lead to underdiagnosis or misinterpretation.

4. **Evolution of Medical Knowledge:** Medical knowledge and understanding of EDS have grown over time. New EDS subtypes have been found, and diagnostic criteria have been improved. Healthcare practitioners may be out of touch with the most recent studies and guidelines.

5. **Misdiagnosis:** EDS is frequently misdiagnosed or diagnosed later in life. Because of the delay in diagnosis, both patients and healthcare providers may be unaware.

6. **Multidisciplinary Approach:** EDS frequently necessitates a multidisciplinary approach including a variety of experts such as rheumatologists, geneticists, orthopedic surgeons, and dermatologists. Collaboration across various medical areas is not always appreciated.

7. **Limited Training Options:** Some medical institutions and training programs may not give comprehensive instruction on uncommon genetic illnesses such as EDS. As a result, healthcare

practitioners may only have limited exposure to such situations during their education.

8. **Patient Advocacy and Awareness:** The EDS community and patient advocacy groups are extremely important in spreading awareness about the illness. The degree of local patient advocacy initiatives may impact the amount of knowledge and support for EDS in some locations.

EDS education for healthcare professionals is being improved, and research on the topic is underway. Individuals with EDS and their families, on the other hand, frequently play an important role in educating their healthcare professionals and advocating for themselves to ensure correct diagnosis and adequate management.

From Uncertainty to Diagnosis: My Journey with Ehlers-Danlos Syndrome

In the early years of motherhood, my days were filled with the simple yet important tasks of caring for my child and maintaining our modest home. However, as my son reached the age to acquire an education, my role expanded to include teaching, and I soon found myself on my feet, guiding him through the intricacies of learning. It was during this time that my life took an unexpected turn.

I had always lived with some level of pain, but as the months went by, my symptoms began to intensify rapidly. Afternoons were no longer opportunities for rest but became a daily ordeal, as I grappled with pain so severe that coherent thought and speech were a challenge. Evenings brought a wave of nausea, and I often found myself bending over the toilet, overwhelmed by the pain. Climbing the stairs at night became a painstaking task that left me exhausted. It was clear that something was amiss, and I decided it was time to seek answers.

I began my search by typing "chronic pain" into the search bar, hoping to find some clarity. I combed through articles, trying to match my symptoms to common causes of neck and back pain. Yet, nothing seemed to fit the agonizing, joint-wrenching pain that I was experiencing.

But then, a moment of clarity struck me like a lightning bolt. I recalled a doctor's visit when I was 19, during which he had asked if anything else was bothering me. I briefly contemplated mentioning the persistent growing pains that had never seemed to go away but ultimately dismissed them as unimportant.

I embarked on a quest to understand these growing pains, and my research led me down a rabbit hole that eventually led me to Ehlers-Danlos Syndrome (EDS). It was as if a puzzle had finally fallen into place, and EDS seemed to account for all of my symptoms.

With a list of diagnostic criteria in hand, I examined myself closely. I wasn't entirely certain if my skin was stretchy enough, but the severe laxity in my joints left no room for doubt.

Armed with the hypothesis that I might have EDS, I delved into the EDS community. There, I learned invaluable lessons in pain management. I taught myself to meditate and practiced unconventional yet effective posture and movement techniques to keep my joints within a more "normal" range of motion.

These homegrown pain management strategies gradually improved my condition. My nightly pain, once a debilitating 7-8 on the pain scale, lessened to a 5-6, allowing me to regain clarity of thought during the day.

It would be years before I received an official diagnosis, primarily due to insurance limitations. However, a pivotal moment came when I was referred to physical therapy and encountered a therapist who shared my connective tissue challenges.

"You have connective tissue disease," she stated.

"But it's not diagnosed," I hesitated.

"I don't have a diagnosed connective tissue disease either," she replied with understanding. At that moment, I realized that our shared experience transcended official labels.

A formal diagnosis eventually followed, initiated by a referral to a rheumatologist. "Suspected Ehlers-Danlos Syndrome" had been my unofficial diagnosis for about a month after my conversation with the physical therapist. My journey, filled with moments of uncertainty and resilience, eventually led me to a diagnosis that provided clarity and a path forward. It was a testament to the power of self-advocacy and the strength that can be found even in the face of chronic pain and medical challenges.

Chapter 2: Symptoms and Clinical Signs

What are the primary symptoms of EDS

Ehlers-Danlos Syndrome (EDS) is a complicated multisystem illness that can cause a variety of symptoms. The major symptoms of EDS differ according to the subtype and person. Below are some of the most common symptoms related to EDS:

1. **Joint Hypermobility:** Many EDS patients have joint hypermobility, which means their joints can move beyond their usual range of motion. This can result in joint discomfort, instability, and a higher chance of dislocations and subluxations.

2. **Skin Abnormalities:** EDS can have a variety of effects on the skin, including:

   - Hyperextensibility of the skin: The skin can be stretched more than normal and may feel smooth and silky.

- Prone to bruising: Due to their weak blood vessels, people with EDS frequently bruise easily.

- Cigarette paper scars: These are thin, atrophic scars that can develop as a result of slight trauma.

3. **Chronic Pain:** Many people with EDS suffer from chronic pain that affects their joints, muscles, and connective tissues. This discomfort can be incapacitating and interfere with normal living.

4. **Joint Dislocations:** Hypermobile joints' instability can lead to repeated joint dislocations and subluxations, producing discomfort and functional restrictions.

5. **Gastrointestinal Symptoms:** EDS can cause gastrointestinal symptoms such as gastritis, reflux, constipation, and abdominal discomfort.

6. **Vascular Issues (in some subtypes):** Vascular EDS (vEDS) is linked to brittle blood vessels and an increased risk of arterial and organ rupture. This is potentially fatal.

7. **Cardiovascular Symptoms (in some subtypes):** Certain subtypes of EDS can cause cardiovascular problems, such as mitral valve prolapse or aortic root dilatation.

8. **Dental and Oral Issues**: EDS can cause problems with the oral cavity, such as dental crowding, high palates, and weak gums.

9. **Fatigue and Weakness:** People with EDS may have chronic tiredness and muscular weakness.

10. **Dysautonomia**: Some people with EDS may have dysautonomia, which can cause symptoms such as fast heartbeat, low blood pressure, and fainting.

11. **Eye Problems:** EDS can affect the eyes, producing myopia (nearsightedness), retinal difficulties, and keratoconus.

12. **Abnormalities in Connective Tissues:** In addition to joints and skin, EDS can damage other connective tissues in the body, such as ligaments, tendons, and blood vessels, resulting in a variety of symptoms.

It's crucial to remember that the degree and mix of these symptoms can vary greatly between EDS patients. Furthermore, because various subtypes of EDS are linked with particular clinical characteristics, symptoms may change between subtypes. For adequate symptom treatment and care, an accurate diagnosis and complete understanding of the subtype are required.

What led to the discovery of EDS

In the early twentieth century, two physicians described and termed Ehlers-Danlos Syndrome (EDS). Here's a timeline of how EDS was discovered and understood:

1. **Historical Observations:** Prior to the formal recognition of EDS, there were historical reports of people with hypermobility, joint instability, and unique skin traits. Some of these accounts extend back centuries, however, the disease was not examined or characterized properly at the time.

2. **Early twentieth century:** In 1901, the Danish dermatologist Edvard Ehlers reported a patient with hypermobility and hyperelasticity of the skin. A few

years later, in 1908, Henri-Alexandre Danlos, a French dermatologist, published a report on a young patient with identical skin and joint features.

3. **Formal Recognition as Ehlers-Danlos Syndrome (EDS):** To recognize the contributions of both Ehlers and Danlos, the disorder was called Ehlers-Danlos Syndrome (EDS). Their findings and publications marked the beginning of the syndrome's formal identification.

4. **Classification and Research:** Over time, researchers and doctors began to identify and classify the many subtypes of EDS based on clinical and genetic variables. The clinical diagnostic criteria were devised and improved.

5. **Genetic Discoveries:** Advances in genetic studies in the late twentieth and early twenty-first centuries resulted in the identification of distinct genetic variants linked to certain EDS subtypes. This has improved knowledge of the syndrome's underlying genetic causes.

6. **Increased Awareness:** As EDS awareness and research have grown, so have diagnostic procedures and management options. Patient advocacy groups and organizations have played an important role in promoting EDS awareness.

While the syndrome was called in the early twentieth century, it required many years of study and genetic developments to get a fuller knowledge of the numerous subtypes, their genetic foundation, and the best strategies for diagnosis and therapy. Ongoing research is critical for improving the lives of people with EDS and advancing our understanding of this complicated disorder.

What effects does EDS have on the skin, joints, and other bodily systems

Ehlers-Danlos Syndrome (EDS) can have a variety of effects on the skin, joints, and other bodily systems, depending on the exact subtype and individual variance.

How EDS can impact different body systems:

1. **Skin:**

- **Skin Hyperextensibility:** Many people with EDS have skin hyperextensibility, which means their skin can be stretched beyond its usual range. This can give the skin a silky and velvety sensation.

- **Easy bruising:** EDS is frequently accompanied by brittle blood vessels, which results in easy bruising. Visible bruises can emerge from minor trauma or strain.

- **Cigarette Paper Scars:** EDS can cause thin, atrophic scars that resemble cigarette paper. These scars might emerge as a result of minor injury or surgery.

- **Thin Skin:** The skin in EDS is frequently thinner than usual, making it more prone to rips and damage.

- **Delayed Wound Healing:** Wounds, particularly surgical wounds, may heal more slowly in people with EDS.

2. Joints:

- Joint Hypermobility: Joint hypermobility is a characteristic shared by numerous EDS subtypes. It indicates that the joints are able to move beyond their usual range of motion, resulting in joint instability, discomfort, and a greater chance of dislocations or subluxations.

- Joint Pain: Chronic joint pain is a common symptom of EDS, and it is generally caused by joint hypermobility and the resulting pressure on the surrounding ligaments and tissues.

- Joint Dislocations: The instability of hypermobile joints can result in recurring joint dislocations and subluxations, adding to discomfort and functional restrictions.

3. Other Body Systems:

- **Cardiovascular System:** Some EDS subtypes can cause problems with the cardiovascular system, such as mitral valve prolapse or aortic root dilatation.

- **Gastrointestinal System:** EDS can produce symptoms such as gastritis, reflux, constipation, and abdominal discomfort.

- **Vascular System (in vEDS):** Vascular EDS (vEDS) is associated with brittle blood vessels, which increases the chance of artery and organ rupture, both of which can be fatal.

- **Muscles and Tendons:** EDS can cause muscular weakening as well as damage to tendons and ligaments, which can contribute to joint instability.

- **Nervous System:** Some people with EDS have dysautonomia, which can cause symptoms including a racing heart, low blood pressure, and fainting.

- **Eyes:** EDS can affect the eyes, causing disorders such as myopia (nearsightedness), retinal issues, and keratoconus.

- **Oral Cavity:** Oral cavity issues, including dental crowding, high palates, and weak gums, can be common in EDS.

It is crucial to remember that the clinical manifestation of EDS varies greatly between persons and subtypes. Furthermore, certain subtypes may have clinical characteristics that others do not. A thorough and accurate diagnosis is essential for customizing therapy and management methods to the unique requirements of people with EDS.

How Symptoms Vary Between Different EDS Types

Because of the various genetic abnormalities associated with each subtype, symptoms of Ehlers-Danlos Syndrome (EDS) can vary dramatically. Here's a summary of how symptoms differ across the many EDS types:

1. **EDS Hypermobility Type (hEDS):**
   - **Primary Symptoms:** Primary symptoms include joint hypermobility, persistent joint

pain, and skin involvement, including skin hyperextensibility and easy bruising.

- **Less Common Problems:** Vascular and organ problems are less common in hEDS than in other subtypes.

2. **Classical EDS (cEDS):**

   - **Primary Symptoms:** Skin hyperextensibility, joint hypermobility, atrophic scarring, and joint instability.

   - **Less Common problems:** In cEDS, severe vascular problems, organ rupture, and muscular hypotonia are less prevalent.

3. **Vascular EDS (vEDS):**

   - **Primary Symptoms:** Fragile blood vessels, higher risk of artery and organ rupture, thin and transparent skin, and joint hypermobility.

   - **Less Common problems:** Vascular problems are the hallmark of vEDS, posing a considerable risk of death. Skin involvement is often minimal.

4. **Kyphoscoliotic EDS (kEDS):**

- **Primary Symptoms:** Severe muscular hypotonia at birth, progressive kyphoscoliosis (a kind of spine curvature), joint hypermobility, and brittle skin.

- **Less Common problems:** In kEDS, joint dislocations and vascular problems are less prevalent.

5. **Arthrochalasia EDS (aEDS):**

- **Primary symptoms:** Severe joint hypermobility, joint dislocations, skin hyperextensibility, and muscular hypotonia are the primary symptoms of Arthrochalasia EDS (aEDS).

- **Less Common problems:** Vascular problems are uncommon in aEDS.

6. **Dermatosparaxis EDS (dEDS):**

- **Primary Symptoms:** Extremely frail and sagging skin, quick bruising, and joint hypermobility.

- **Less Common problems:** Vascular and organ problems are rare in dEDS.

7. **Brittle Cornea Syndrome (BCS):**

   - **Primary Symptoms: Primary symptoms** include thin and easily torn corneas (the clear front area of the eye), joint hypermobility, and fragile skin.

   - **Less Common problems:** Vascular and organ problems are uncommon in BCS.

8. **Musculocontractural EDS (mcEDS):**

   - **Primary Characteristics:** Congenital muscular weakness, joint contractures, unique facial traits, and skin involvement.

   - **Less Common problems:** Vascular and organ problems are rare with mcEDS.

While these descriptions emphasize some key and less frequent traits, it is crucial to remember that EDS is a very varied disorder. Individuals with the same subtype may have a variety of symptoms and severity. Furthermore, because some EDS subtypes are uncommon, they are less well-known than the more prevalent forms. Accurate diagnosis and a multidisciplinary approach to care are required to customize therapy and management to the specific needs of each individual.

Uncommon and Unusual Symptoms

In addition to the major symptoms of Ehlers-Danlos Syndrome (EDS), individuals with EDS may develop less common or unusual symptoms. These symptoms can differ across EDS subtypes and people. Among the less frequent or unusual symptoms are:

1. **Gastrointestinal Problems:** EDS can cause a variety of gastrointestinal issues, including gastritis, reflux, constipation, and abdominal discomfort. These concerns may be less evident at times but can have a substantial influence on an individual's quality of life.

2. **Dental and Oral Issues:** EDS patients may have dental crowding, high palates, and weak gums. These dental and oral concerns can cause dental pain and oral hygiene problems.

3. **Nervous System Involvement:** Some people with EDS may suffer from dysautonomia, a malfunction of the autonomic nerve system that causes symptoms such as fast heartbeat, low blood pressure, and fainting. This is less common but more significant.

4. **Chronic Fatigue:** Although chronic tiredness is a typical symptom of EDS, its degree varies. Some people have significant exhaustion that interferes with their everyday functioning, while others have more acceptable degrees of fatigue.

5. **Dysphasia:** Individuals with EDS may encounter difficulties swallowing or speaking in some circumstances due to muscle and connective tissue involvement.

6. **Eye Issues:** EDS can have a variety of effects on the eyes, including the development of myopia (nearsightedness), retinal difficulties, and keratoconus (a corneal issue). These eye-related symptoms are less prevalent, but they should be closely examined.

7. **Mood and Mental Health:** Chronic pain and physical restrictions can have a negative impact on mental health. Depression, anxiety, and other mood problems are less prevalent but crucial elements of EDS.

8. **Cardiovascular Issues (in some subtypes):** Cardiovascular issues, such as mitral valve prolapse or aortic root dilatation, are more likely in specific subtypes of EDS, such as classical and hypermobility EDS.

9. **Organ Complications (in others Subtypes):** While organ complications are uncommon in many EDS subtypes, others, such as vascular EDS (vEDS), are linked with a significant risk of organ rupture and internal hemorrhage, both of which can be fatal.

10. **Neurological Symptoms:** Some people with EDS may develop neurological symptoms such as headaches, nerve compression, and nerve pain, especially if the spine or nerves are involved.

These less common or unusual symptoms might vary greatly between people and are not always present in cases with EDS. Because of the condition's complexity and diversity, a thorough approach to diagnosis and management is required to accommodate the unique demands and problems that each individual with EDS faces.

The Risks Associated With Eds

Ehlers-Danlos Syndrome (EDS) can cause a variety of problems, which vary based on the subtype of EDS and individual circumstances. Some of the probable consequences of EDS are as follows:

1. **Joint Complications:**
   - Frequent joint dislocations and subluxations can result in chronic joint discomfort and functional limitations;
   - Osteoarthritis may develop over time in afflicted joints.
2. **Skin Complications:**

- Fragile skin can cause bruises, skin tears, and poor wound healing.
- Scarring can worsen, including atrophic or "cigarette paper" scars.

3. Chronic Pain:

- Persistent and widespread pain can have a substantial impact on an individual's quality of life.

4. Cardiovascular Issues (in certain subtypes):

- Vascular EDS (vEDS) is linked with a significant risk of artery rupture, organ rupture, and internal hemorrhage, all of which can be fatal.
- Mitral valve prolapse and aortic root dilatation may occur in some EDS subtypes.

5. Gastrointestinal Complications:

- Gastritis, reflux, constipation, and stomach discomfort can all have an influence on the digestive system, affecting nutrition and general well-being.

6. **Dental and Oral Issues:**

- Dental crowding, high palates, and weak gums can cause dental pain and oral hygiene issues.

7. **Dysautonomia:**

- Dysautonomia, which affects the autonomic nerve system, can cause symptoms such as fast heart rate, low blood pressure, and fainting.

8. **Neurological Symptoms:**

- EDS can cause neurological symptoms such as headaches, nerve compression, and nerve discomfort, especially in situations involving the spine or nerves.

9. **Gynecological and Obstetric difficulties:**

- Women with EDS may face pregnancy and delivery difficulties, such as increased joint laxity and the possibility of birth canal or uterine abnormalities.

10. Mood and Mental Health Issues:

- Living with chronic pain and physical restrictions can have an influence on mental health, leading to illnesses such as sadness and anxiety.

11. Eye Complications:

- Vision can be affected by eye diseases such as myopia, retinal difficulties, and keratoconus.

12. Muscle Weakness and Fatigue:

- Muscle weakness can limit physical activity, and persistent weariness can interfere with everyday functioning.

13. Organ Prolapse:

- Some people with EDS may suffer from organ prolapse, such as pelvic organ prolapse or rectal prolapse.

It's vital to remember that the severity of these issues varies between people and EDS subtypes. Proper treatment, early diagnosis, and medical care are critical to reducing the risk of problems and improving the quality of life for those with EDS. A multidisciplinary strategy including several medical professionals may be required depending on the degree of treatment.

Nutrition for EDS patients

Nutrition is unquestionably important in the therapy of Ehlers-Danlos Syndrome (EDS). A well-balanced diet can aid with particular EDS problems including inflammation, collagen formation, and general health. Here's a thorough food and nutrition advice for EDS patients:

Dietary Guidelines for EDS Patients

1. **Foods that are anti-inflammatory:** Chronic pain and inflammation are frequently associated with EDS. Include anti-inflammatory foods like fruits (berries, cherries), vegetables (leafy greens, broccoli), fatty fish (salmon, mackerel), nuts (walnuts, almonds), and spices (turmeric, ginger) in your diet.

2. **Collagen-Boosting Nutrients:** Collagen deficiency is a hallmark of EDS. Consume collagen-promoting nutrients such as vitamin C (found in citrus fruits, strawberries, and peppers), proline (found in dairy products, eggs, and meat), and glycine (found in bone broth, chicken skin, and pork skin).

3. **Hydration:** Proper hydration is critical for joint health and skin elasticity. Drink plenty of water throughout the day. Herbal teas and infused water can be refreshing.

4. **Balanced Diet:** To promote general health and energy levels, maintain a balanced diet that contains a mix of macronutrients (carbohydrates, proteins, and healthy fats).

5. **Vitamin and Mineral Supplements:** Depending on your EDS type and symptoms, you may require vitamin and mineral supplements, notably vitamin D, calcium, and magnesium for bone health. Consult a healthcare practitioner for specific advice.

6. **Protein Sources:** Lean proteins, such as poultry, fish, tofu, and lentils, can aid with muscle and joint stability.

7. **Omega-3 Fatty Acids:** Found in fatty fish, flaxseeds, and walnuts, these fats have anti-inflammatory qualities and can aid in the management of pain and inflammation.

8. **Fiber:** A diet high in fiber from whole grains, fruits, and vegetables can help with digestion, which is frequently an issue for persons with EDS.

9. **Avoid Trigger Foods:** Recognize and avoid foods that may cause inflammation, allergies, or digestive problems. Because this varies from person to person, maintaining a food diary may be beneficial.

Meal Preparation and Eating Habits

1. **Small, Frequent Meals:** EDS patients may struggle with joint and muscular stability, which can interfere with meal preparation. To lessen the physical strain of cooking and eating, consider eating smaller, more often meals.

2. **Food Preparation:** Use kitchen equipment and tools like food processors and jar openers to make meal preparation easier.

3. **Chewing and Swallowing:** If you have trouble with your jaw stability, choose softer meals or blended choices like smoothies and soups.

Digestive Health

1. **Probiotics:** To maintain gut health, consume probiotic-rich foods (yogurt, kefir, sauerkraut) or take a probiotic supplement.
2. **Low-Residue Diet:** If you suffer from gastrointestinal problems, a low-residue diet that restricts high-fiber foods may be useful.

Consult a Medical Professional

EDS patients must collaborate with a healthcare specialist, such as a dietitian or nutritionist, to develop a specific dietary plan. They can assist you in customizing your diet to your individual EDS type and symptoms. They can also evaluate your nutritional condition and, if necessary, offer suitable supplements.

Remember that diet is an important element of controlling EDS, but it should be part of a comprehensive plan that includes adequate medical care, physical therapy, and emotional support.

Eating for Energy and Pain Management

1. **Balanced Carbohydrates:** For a constant supply of energy, choose complex carbs such as whole grains, lentils, and starchy vegetables. Spreading your carbohydrate consumption throughout the day might aid with energy maintenance.

2. **Hydration Strategies:** It is critical to stay hydrated because dehydration can increase symptoms. Some EDS patients may have swallowing or proprioception difficulties, making drinking difficult. Drinking water throughout the day or using a straw might be beneficial.

3. **Supplemental Shakes:** In circumstances where chewing and digestion are difficult, nutritional supplement shakes or drinks that supply necessary nutrients in a more readily digested form may be considered.

Foods to Avoid

1. **Processed Foods:** Limit or avoid highly processed meals, which typically include additives, artificial

preservatives, and high quantities of salt, all of which can aggravate inflammation.

2. **High-Glycemic and Sugary Foods:** These might cause blood sugar spikes and crashes, thereby exacerbating exhaustion and discomfort.

3. **Caffeine and alcohol:** These drugs can disrupt sleep, cause dehydration, and lead to inflammation in some people. Moderation is essential.

4. **High-salt Foods:** Too much salt can cause water retention and aggravate joint-related discomfort. Choose low-sodium options.

5. **Food allergies:** Identify and avoid any food allergies or sensitivities that may aggravate inflammation or gastrointestinal symptoms.

Customized Nutrition Plan

Keep in mind that the effects of EDS might differ greatly from person to person. As a result, it's critical to develop a personalized dietary plan in collaboration with a healthcare physician or nutritionist. They may assist you in addressing your unique needs, tracking your progress, and adjusting your diet as needed.

Finally, while diet is important in controlling EDS, it is only one component of a comprehensive treatment plan. A comprehensive strategy that combines correct medical treatment, physical therapy, and emotional support is required for optimal EDS management. Maintaining an open line of contact with healthcare providers is also essential for making educated decisions regarding your dietary and nutritional requirements.

Meal-Planning Tips

Here are some meal-planning suggestions geared exclusively for those with Ehlers-Danlos Syndrome (EDS):

1. Consult a Registered Dietician:

- Seek advice from a registered dietician who is familiar with EDS. They can assist you in developing a customized food plan depending on your individual kind of EDS, symptoms, and dietary limitations.

2. Maintain a Healthy Nutrient Balance:

- Make sure your meals contain a variety of macronutrients, such as carbs, proteins, and healthy fats.

- Include a variety of foods to ensure adequate vitamin and mineral intake.

- Concentrate on anti-inflammatory foods like fruits and vegetables, lean meats, and whole grains.

3. Regular Eating Routine:

- Plan frequent meals and snacks throughout the day to keep your energy levels steady.

- This can assist in avoiding energy dumps and joint strain caused by overexertion while hungry.

4. Hydration:

- Keep hydrated to preserve tissue elasticity and general health. Water is the greatest option, although herbal teas and diluted fruit juices can also help you stay hydrated.

5. Small, Frequent Meals:

- Smaller, more frequent meals may be simpler to digest for persons suffering from EDS-related gastrointestinal difficulties.

- Avoid heavy, big meals, which might cause pain or stomach issues.

6. Mindful Eating:

- Eat carefully and pay heed to your body's suggestions. Chewing your meal completely can aid digestion while also reducing joint pain.

- Pay attention to your body's hunger and fullness signals.

7. Food Diary:

- Maintain a food journal to document how various foods impact your symptoms. This can assist you in identifying trigger foods and improving your dietary choices.

8. Plan ahead of time:

- Plan your meals and snacks ahead of time, and think about batch cooking for ease.

- Meal preparation ahead of time lowers the physical strain of regular cooking.

9. Stock EDS-Friendly Foods:

- Keep items that are easy to prepare and mild on your digestion in your kitchen. Soft fruits, lean meats, and readily digested cereals may be included.

10. Sensitivity Temperature:

- Individuals with EDS who are temperature sensitive may find hot or cold meals unpleasant. Choose items that are at a moderate temperature, or let spicy foods cool somewhat before consuming.

11. Supplementation:

- If you're having trouble achieving your nutritional needs via diet alone, talk to your doctor about the need for particular supplements like vitamins and minerals.

12. Joint-Friendly Cooking Techniques:

- Slow cooking, steaming, or poaching are all good ways to make meals softer and easier to chew.

- Reduce the amount of rough or chewy meals that might strain your jaw and muscular joints.

13. Limit Sugar and Processed Foods:

- Sugary snacks and processed meals, which can aggravate inflammation and cause energy dumps, should be limited or avoided.

14. Listen to Your Body:

- Be aware of how your body reacts to different meals and change your diet appropriately.

- Don't be afraid to seek assistance on nutrition management from your dietician or healthcare practitioner.

Remember that meal planning should be flexible and tailored to your own requirements. Through your food choices, you want to improve your general health, control EDS-related symptoms, and promote well-being.

Chapter 3: Management and Treatment

How To Managed Eds on a Day-To-Day Basis

On a daily level, Ehlers-Danlos Syndrome (EDS) care often entails a variety of measures to alleviate symptoms and enhance quality of life. Here are some major features of EDS management:

1. Medical Care and Monitoring:

- It is critical to have regular medical check-ups in order to monitor and manage the disease.
- Ongoing care may require specialized healthcare providers such as rheumatologists, geneticists, physical therapists, and pain specialists.

2. Pain Management:

- Chronic pain is a frequent EDS symptom. Medication, physical therapy, and other techniques may be used to treat pain.

- Physical therapy can aid in the stabilization of joints, the improvement of muscular strength, and the management of pain.

3. Assistive Devices:

- The use of assistive devices such as braces, splints, and orthotics can give joint support and stability.
- In certain circumstances, mobility assistance such as canes or wheelchairs may be required.

4. Lifestyle Modifications:

- Lifestyle modifications, such as timing activities and avoiding overexertion, can help prevent joint issues.
- Adequate rest and sleep are essential for tiredness management.

5. Exercise and Rehabilitation:

- Individualized exercise regimens can help strengthen muscles, promote joint stability, and improve general fitness.
- Low-impact workouts and aquatic treatment are frequently advised.

6. Dietary and Nutritional Support:

- Eating a well-balanced diet rich in collagen-boosting elements such as vitamin C can help.

- In certain circumstances, nutritional supplementation may be recommended.

7. Psychological and Emotional Support:

- Mental health assistance is crucial to address the emotional burden of living with EDS.

- Cognitive-behavioral therapy and stress management approaches can be beneficial.

8. Medications:

- Medications may be administered to treat particular symptoms such as pain, gastrointestinal problems, or cardiovascular difficulties.

- In some EDS subtypes, blood pressure medicines are used to treat autonomic dysfunction.

9. Surgery:

- Surgery is considered on an individual basis for conditions such as joint instability or organ difficulties.

- Because of the higher risk of complications with EDS, more attention is required while planning procedures.

10. Genetic Counseling:

- Genetic counseling can give information on inheritance patterns and the risk of transferring EDS to future generations to people with EDS and their families.

11. Patient Education:

- Individuals and their families must be educated about EDS. Understanding the illness can aid in the management of symptoms and the avoidance of potential problems.

12. Supportive Communities:

- Support groups and patient advocacy organizations may give useful information, emotional support, and a feeling of community to those with EDS.

Managing EDS on a daily basis frequently necessitates a tailored strategy that takes into account the specific subtype, the severity of symptoms, and the individual's unique requirements and aspirations. Collaboration with healthcare experts, attention to medical guidance, and self-care practices are all critical components in managing EDS effectively.

Treatment options for EDS-related pain and joint instability

To successfully manage the pain and joint instability associated with Ehlers-Danlos Syndrome (EDS), therapy options often entail a multidisciplinary approach. Below are some of the most important therapy options:

1. **Physical Therapy:**

- Physical therapy is an essential component of EDS care. A physical therapist can design a specific exercise program to increase joint stability, muscular strength, and pain relief.
- To treat pain and enhance joint health, therapeutic techniques such as heat, ice, and manual therapy may be employed.

2. Assistive Devices:

- Orthotic equipment, such as braces, splints, and orthopedic shoes, can give support and stability to hypermobile joints.

- Mobility aids such as canes or wheelchairs may be required to alleviate joint strain and avoid falls.

3. Medications:

- Over-the-counter pain remedies such as acetaminophen or nonsteroidal anti-inflammatory drugs (NSAIDs) may help control mild to moderate pain.

- For more severe pain, prescription medications such as muscle relaxants or opioids may be recommended. Opioids, on the other hand, are normally avoided or taken with caution because of the potential for addiction and hyperalgesia.

4. Joint Protection Strategies:

- Learning joint protection strategies, such as bracing or taping, can assist patients with EDS in avoiding overstretching or hyperextending their joints.

5. Strengthening Exercises:

- Specific workouts to strengthen the muscles around hypermobile joints might give additional support and stability.

- Because of its low-impact nature, aquatic treatment, in particular, can be useful for those with EDS.

6. Pain Management Techniques:

- Techniques such as heat or cold therapy, transcutaneous electrical nerve stimulation (TENS), and acupuncture can assist control of pain.

7. Lifestyle Modifications:

- Pacing activities, taking frequent pauses, and avoiding overexertion can help prevent injury and weariness.

- Maintaining a balanced diet and appropriate water can help with general health.

8. Psychological Support:

- Coping with chronic pain and the impact of EDS on daily life may need psychological help. Cognitive behavioral therapy and stress management approaches can both be beneficial.

9. Surgery (in selected cases):

- Surgical procedures may be explored in situations with significant joint instability or consequences such as torn ligaments. Surgery in EDS, on the other hand, can be difficult and risky, thus it is carefully reviewed and treated.

10. Genetic Counseling:

- Genetic counseling can offer information on the risk of passing EDS on to future generations and assist individuals in making educated family planning decisions.

Treatment regimens for EDS-related pain and joint instability should be tailored to each individual's needs, taking into account the EDS subtype, symptom intensity, and impact on daily life. Physical therapists, pain specialists, and orthopedic surgeons may work together as part of a multidisciplinary healthcare team to establish and implement the most effective treatment plan for each patient.

Preventative measures to consider

Individuals with Ehlers-Danlos Syndrome (EDS) can benefit from preventative steps to assist them in managing their disease and lower the risk of complications.

1. Joint Protection:

- Learn joint protection measures to reduce the likelihood of joint dislocations or subluxations. Bracing, taping, or preventing hyperextension are examples of these strategies.

2. Physical Therapy and Exercise:

- Participate in physical therapy and exercises designed to strengthen muscles and improve joint stability on a regular basis.

- Low-impact exercises such as swimming and aquatic therapy can be very effective.

3. Lifestyle Changes:

- Pace your activities to minimize overexertion and weariness.

- Support susceptible joints using assistive devices such as braces or orthotics.

4. Avoid High-Risk Activities:

- Exercise caution while engaging in activities that have a high risk of injury or joint strain. Avoid or modify actions that may result in damage.

5. Hydration and Nutrition:

- To promote general health, maintain sufficient hydration and a balanced diet.

- Getting enough collagen-boosting foods, such as vitamin C, may help.

6. Fall Prevention:

- Take care to avoid falls that might result in joint damage. Maintain a safe living environment and, if necessary, employ mobility aids.

7. Psychological Support:

- Seek psychological treatment and stress management skills to help you cope with the emotional effects of chronic pain and physical limitations.

8. Regular Medical Check-ups:

- Schedule frequent medical check-ups with healthcare experts who are familiar with EDS to monitor the condition and manage any emergent difficulties.

9. Genetic Counseling:

- Consider genetic counseling to better understand inheritance patterns and the possibility of passing EDS on to future generations.

10. Medication Safety:

- Follow recommended dosages and check with healthcare experts about potential interactions and adverse effects, especially if using medication to manage pain.

11. **Surgery Precautions:**

- If surgery is required, discuss your EDS diagnosis with your surgical team. To lessen the risk of problems, special attention and measures may be required.

Preventive treatments should be tailored to the specific EDS subtype, the severity of symptoms, and the individual's demands and lifestyle. Working with a healthcare team that includes EDS specialists can assist patients in developing a specific plan for preventive and symptom management.

Role of Physical Therapy in eds Management

Physical therapy is essential in the treatment of Ehlers-Danlos Syndrome (EDS). It is an important part of treatment because it may assist people with EDS in addressing joint instability, managing pain, and enhancing their overall quality of life. The following are the major functions that physical therapy plays in the management of EDS:

1. **Strengthening and Stabilizing Joints:**

- Physical therapists create exercise programs that are tailored to the individual's specific needs, with a focus on strengthening the muscles surrounding hypermobile joints.

- Strengthening these muscles can provide additional support to the joints, reducing the risk of dislocations or subluxations.

2. **Improving Joint Stability:**

- Physical therapy tries to enhance joint stability and proprioception, which is the body's understanding of its own location. This can assist people with EDS in acquiring control of their hypermobile joints.

3. **Pain Management:**

- Therapists utilize a number of pain management approaches, such as manual therapy, stretching, and therapeutic modalities such as heat and cold therapy.

- Physical therapy can help to alleviate the pain and suffering associated with EDS.

4. Joint Protection:

- Physical therapists educate people with EDS on joint protection strategies to prevent overextension and hyperextension.

- Taping and bracing techniques may be advised to offer additional support.

5. Functional Improvement:

- Physical therapy can improve functional capacities such as walking, standing, and completing activities of daily life. This allows people with EDS to preserve their independence.

6. Postural Training:

- EDS can have an impact on posture owing to joint instability. Physical therapists seek to improve posture and body mechanics in order to alleviate joint and muscle strain.

7. Hypermobility Management:

- Physical therapists give techniques for controlling hypermobile joints and avoiding joint injuries for persons with joint hypermobility.

8. Exercise Guidelines:

- Physical therapists provide exercise guidelines, including recommendations for low-impact exercises and aquatic treatment, which are appropriate for people with EDS.

9. Progress Monitoring:

- Therapy progress is regularly evaluated in order to assess improvements and change treatment programs as appropriate.
- Physical therapists may work with other members of the healthcare team to ensure that patients receive complete treatment.

10. Education:

- Education is a critical component of EDS physical therapy. Individuals with EDS and their families benefit from therapists' knowledge of the disorder, symptom treatment, and injury prevention measures.

Physical therapy is a common element of EDS treatment. Physical therapists can help people maintain joint health, manage pain, and enhance function on a regular basis. Physical therapy exercises and procedures are tailored to the individual's specific needs and EDS subtype, assuring safe and successful condition treatment.

The significance of lifestyle changes and self-care

Individuals suffering from Ehlers-Danlos Syndrome (EDS) must prioritize lifestyle changes and self-care. These measures are crucial in controlling the disease, enhancing quality of life, and avoiding complications. Here are some of the reasons why lifestyle changes and self-care are so important for people with EDS:

1. Symptom Management: EDS can cause a variety of symptoms such as joint instability, persistent discomfort, exhaustion, and skin fragility.

Individuals can effectively control these symptoms by making lifestyle changes and using self-care practices.

2. Joint Protection: Due to joint hypermobility, people with EDS are more likely to suffer joint dislocations and subluxations. Joint injuries can be avoided by learning joint protection measures such as bracing and avoiding overextension.

3. Preventing consequences: EDS can result in a variety of consequences, including skin rips, dental troubles, and cardiovascular concerns. Self-care and lifestyle changes can help avoid or reduce these issues, hence improving overall health.

4. Quality of Life: Individuals with EDS can improve their quality of life by adopting lifestyle adjustments and practicing self-care. Managing pain, minimizing the frequency of joint dislocations, and preserving physical and mental well-being are all part of this.

5. Empowerment and Independence: Empowering people with EDS via self-care education allows

them to take an active part in their condition management. This might provide them with more freedom and control over their health.

6. Fall Prevention: EDS can increase the chance of falling, resulting in joint damage. Individuals can lower their risk of falling by providing a safe living environment, employing assistive equipment, and following good mobility practices.

7. Emotional Well-Being: Living with a chronic disease such as EDS can have a negative impact on one's emotional health. Maintaining emotional well-being requires self-care practices, stress management, and psychological assistance.

8. Health Maintenance: EDS can have an impact on several bodily systems. Individuals may better manage their general health and lower the risk of difficulties by eating a balanced diet, staying hydrated, and getting regular medical check-ups.

9. Avoiding Overexertion: Overexertion might aggravate EDS-related tiredness. Adjustments to one's lifestyle, such as timing activities and

allowing for enough rest, can assist in managing fatigue.

10. Long-Term perspective: Self-care and lifestyle changes help to improve one's long-term perspective. They can aid in the maintenance of an individual's health and well-being, perhaps delaying the growth of certain symptoms or consequences.

11. Collaboration with Healthcare professionals: Individuals can work more successfully with their healthcare professionals to establish and implement tailored treatment programs if they actively participate in self-care and make lifestyle changes.

lifestyle changes and self-care are critical components of EDS treatment. These measures can result in better symptom management, a lower risk of complications, and an overall higher quality of life. Individuals with EDS can improve their well-being and manage their condition by taking an active part in self-care.

STRENGTHENING EXERCISES

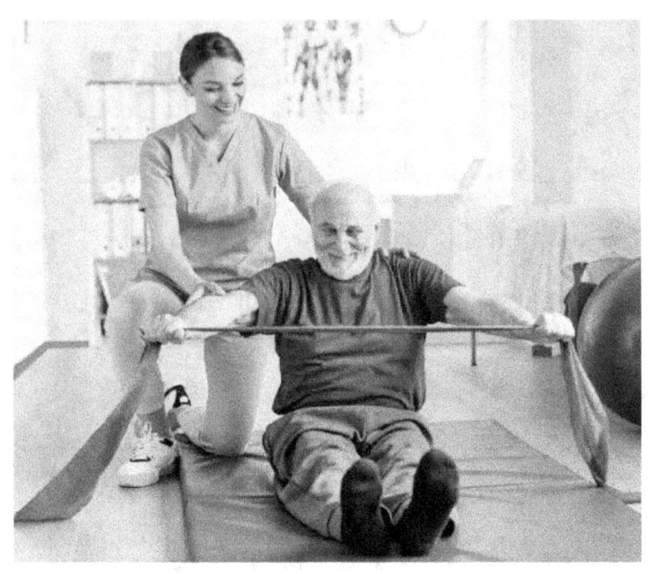

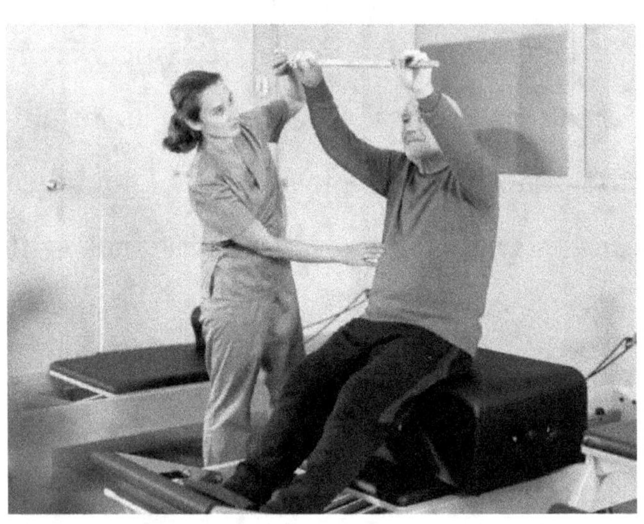

Chapter 4: Living with EDS: Emotional and Psychological Aspects

How EDS impact the emotional and mental well-being of patients

Ehlers-Danlos Syndrome (EDS) has a significant influence on patients' emotional and psychological well-being. Living with a chronic and sometimes invisible ailment may be emotionally taxing, and EDS adds to the mix. Here's how EDS can impair patients' emotional and mental well-being:

1. **Chronic Pain:** Many people with EDS suffer from chronic pain, which may be both physically and emotionally taxing. Coping with chronic pain can result in irritation, sadness, and worry.

2. **Uncertainty:** EDS is a complicated and varied disease. The unpredictability of symptom development, the possibility of complications, and

the absence of a solution can all contribute to severe worry and stress.

3. **The Diagnosis Journey:** Obtaining an EDS diagnosis may be a time-consuming and difficult process. Patients may experience skepticism from healthcare personnel, as well as misdiagnoses and a lack of comprehension, which can lead to frustration and feelings of dismissal.

4. **Social Isolation:** Because some people with EDS have limited movement and energy, they may become socially isolated. Loneliness and sadness can be exacerbated by feeling cut off from friends and loved ones.

5. **Loss of Independence:** Joint instability and physical restrictions caused by EDS can lead to a loss of independence. It might be emotionally challenging to adjust to a more reliant lifestyle.

6. **Body Image and Self-Esteem:** Due to skin fragility and scarring, EDS can have an impact on physical appearance. This can have an impact on one's body

image and self-esteem, perhaps leading to emotions of self-consciousness and self-worth.

7. **Coping with Flare-Ups:** EDS frequently causes symptom flare-ups, which cause symptoms to temporarily intensify. Coping with these erratic bouts can be emotionally draining.

8. **Concern about consequences:** Certain EDS subtypes, such as vascular EDS, are associated with a significant risk of life-threatening consequences. The continual concern of serious health problems can cause anxiety and mental discomfort.

9. **Mental Health Issues:** Because of the tension and suffering associated with the illness, people with EDS may be predisposed to mental health issues such as depression and anxiety.

10. **Emotional Resilience:** Many people with EDS exhibit extraordinary emotional resilience, adaptability, and tenacity in the face of hardship. They frequently become advocates for themselves as well as the EDS community.

11. **Support Systems:** It is critical for emotional well-being to have a solid support system, which may include friends, family, support groups, and mental health specialists. These networks offer comprehension, confirmation, and encouragement.

12. **Coping Strategies:** Learning appropriate coping methods, such as stress management and mindfulness, can assist individuals in navigating the emotional challenges of EDS.

13. **Advocacy and Education:** Learning about EDS and advocating for oneself may empower people and improve their emotional well-being.

14. **Professional Mental Health help:** Seeking professional mental health help, such as therapy and counseling, can give strategies for dealing with the emotional effects of EDS.

It is critical to recognize the emotional and psychological elements of EDS and to offer comprehensive care that addresses not just physical symptoms but also the emotional needs of those living with the illness. A comprehensive strategy that includes physical and mental well-being is critical for improving EDS sufferers' overall quality of life.

Good coping methods that are beneficial for people with EDS

Coping with Ehlers-Danlos Syndrome (EDS) can be difficult, but there are a number of useful coping methods that people with EDS can use to manage the disease and improve their quality of life. Here are some useful coping skills for people with EDS:

1. Pain Management:

- Work with your healthcare professionals to build a pain management strategy that is personalized to your individual requirements. Medication, physical therapy, and other pain treatment approaches may be included in this regimen.

2. Physical Therapy and Exercise:

- Participate in frequent physical therapy and exercise programs designed to strengthen muscles, improve joint stability, and reduce discomfort.

3. Joint Protection:

- Learn joint protection measures to reduce the likelihood of joint dislocations or subluxations. Bracing, taping, or changing daily routines are examples of these strategies.

4. Stress Management:

- Reduce the emotional effect of living with a chronic disease by using stress management strategies such as deep breathing, mindfulness, and meditation.

5. Supportive Communities:

- Connect with EDS support groups or patient advocacy organizations to exchange experiences, learn knowledge, and get emotional support.

6. Psychological Support:

- Seek professional mental health help, such as therapy or counseling, to address the emotional issues associated with EDS.

7. Self-Care:

- Make self-care habits that enhance physical and emotional well-being a priority. This involves getting enough rest, eating healthy food, and keeping a positive atmosphere.

8. Assistive Devices:

- Use supportive devices such as braces, splints, or mobility aids to increase joint stability and minimize strain.

9. Mobility and Fall Prevention:

- Make changes to your living environment to reduce falls and injuries, such as adding handrails or using non-slip mats. Take precautions and keep your mobility in mind.

10. **Pain Journal**:

- Keep a pain notebook to record symptoms, triggers, and pain patterns. This can assist healthcare experts in better understanding your situation and revising your treatment approach.

11. Goal Setting:

- Set attainable short-term and long-term objectives to retain motivation and a feeling of purpose.

12. Concentrate on Your strengths:

- Rather than obsessing over your limits, concentrate on your strengths and what you can achieve.

13. Stay Informed:

- Learn about EDS from credible sources and medical specialists. Individuals with knowledge are better able to make educated decisions regarding their health care.

13. Adapt and Modify Activities:

- Adapt regular activities to your condition. Prioritize activities that will not aggravate your EDS symptoms.

Remember that coping tactics differ from person to person, and it's critical to adjust these strategies to your personal requirements and EDS subtype. A multidisciplinary approach to treatment that includes collaboration with healthcare practitioners as well as assistance from friends and family can be very successful in assisting those with EDS to manage the condition's problems.

Approaches to aid patients and their families in comprehending and handling potential difficulties.

Understanding and treating the issues associated with Ehlers-Danlos Syndrome (EDS) necessitates proactive efforts on the part of both patients and their families. Patients and families can take the following actions to better understand and manage the issues connected with EDS:

1. Education:

- Learn as much as possible about EDS. To learn more about the disorder, its subtypes, and management techniques, consult credible sources such as medical specialists, EDS groups, and trusted websites.

2. Maintain Open and Honest Communication:

- Maintain open and honest communication within the family. To encourage awareness and emotional support, share your views, worries, and experiences with EDS.

3. Healthcare Team:

- Create a robust healthcare team comprised of professionals knowledgeable with EDS. Consult with them on a regular basis to treat symptoms and obtain specialized care.

4. Support Groups:

- Join EDS support groups or communities in person or online to connect with people who have had similar experiences. These organizations offer invaluable emotional support as well as a forum for information exchange.

5. Support for Mental Health:

- Consider counseling or therapy for both patients and family members. Living with a chronic disease may be emotionally draining, therefore professional mental health help can be quite useful.

6. Self-Advocacy:

- Encourage patients to become their own advocates. This entails being proactive in their healthcare, asking questions, and obtaining second opinions when necessary.

7. Lifestyle Adjustments:

- Work together to make required lifestyle changes to fit the requirements of the individual with EDS. This may include adjustments to the living environment, food changes, and exercise regimens.

8. Caregiver Education:

- Make certain that family members who serve as caregivers are knowledgeable about EDS and its management. They should be aware of the patient's limits, help with everyday duties, and offer emotional support.

9. Goal Setting:

- Establish realistic short-term and long-term goals. Individuals with EDS may be motivated to maintain a feeling of purpose and focus on good accomplishments as a result of this.

10. Collaborative Care:

- Encourage teamwork among healthcare professionals to ensure EDS patients receive complete care. Multidisciplinary teams can handle the condition's different elements.

11. Patience and Empathy:

- Exercise patience and empathy. EDS symptoms can vary, and individuals might have good and poor days. Understand and accept their limits without passing judgment.

12. Encourage Independence:

- Encourage people with EDS to preserve their independence to the best of their abilities. This boosts self-esteem and gives them a sense of control over their life.

13. Respite Care:

- Consider possibilities for caregiver respite care. Caring for a loved one who has a chronic illness may be taxing, and respite care can bring a much-needed break.

14. Emergency Plan:

- Create an emergency plan outlining how to respond in the event of acute EDS problems. This plan should be shared with family members, caregivers, and healthcare practitioners.

15. Raise Awareness:

- Raise EDS awareness in your neighborhood and social networks. This can assist in reducing stigma, increasing understanding, and gaining support.

16. Recognize Achievements:

- Recognize small and huge accomplishments since they contribute to a happy mentality and emotional well-being.

Understanding and managing the problems of EDS is a continuous effort involving education, communication, and a proactive approach to treatment. Patients and their families can improve their overall quality of life by working together as a team to cope with the disease.

Available resources and support networks for EDS patients

Patients with Ehlers-Danlos Syndrome (EDS) have access to a range of tools and support networks that may give vital knowledge, emotional support, and connections with others who have had similar symptoms. Bellow are some of the most important websites and support networks for EDS patients:

1. Ehlers-Danlos Support Organizations:

- Organizations like the Ehlers-Danlos Society and national EDS organizations provide a wealth of information on EDS, research updates, and resources for patients and their families.

2. Support Groups:

- Local and online support groups bring together individuals with EDS to share their experiences, challenges, and coping strategies. These groups offer a sense of community and emotional support.

3. Patient Advocacy Groups:

- Patient advocacy groups, such as the EDS Awareness and Support Group, focus on raising awareness, supporting patients, and advocating for better medical care and research.

4. Social Media Communities:

- EDS-related groups and communities on social media platforms like Facebook, Instagram, and Twitter provide opportunities to connect with others, ask questions, and access shared resources.

5. Medical Professionals:

- Rheumatologists, geneticists, and other specialists with expertise in EDS are valuable resources for medical guidance, treatment, and management strategies.

6. EDS Clinics and Centers:

- Some healthcare institutions have specialized EDS clinics or centers where patients can receive comprehensive care from a multidisciplinary team.

7. Online Resources:

- Reputable websites, such as the Ehlers-Danlos Society's website, offer a wide range of information, from EDS subtypes and diagnostic criteria to treatment guidelines.

8. EDS Publications and Newsletters:

- EDS-specific publications and newsletters, such as "The Ehlers-Danlos Times," provide updates on research, personal stories, and community events.

9. Educational Events:

- Attend conferences, seminars, and webinars on EDS to gain knowledge, connect with experts, and meet other individuals living with the condition.

10. Therapists and Counselors: - Mental health professionals can offer emotional support, coping strategies, and stress management techniques to help patients and their families address the emotional aspects of EDS.

11. Genetic Counselors: - Genetic counselors can provide information on the inheritance pattern of EDS and offer guidance for family planning and genetic testing.

12. Rare Disease Networks: - Rare disease networks, such as the National Organization for Rare Disorders (NORD), can provide resources and advocacy for individuals with EDS.

13. Caregiver Support Groups: - Caregiver support groups offer emotional support and resources for family members and friends who provide care for individuals with EDS.

14. Books and Literature: - Books written by medical professionals and individuals with EDS can provide in-depth information on the condition, treatment options, and personal experiences.

15. Assistive Device Suppliers: - Suppliers of assistive devices, such as braces and mobility aids, can help individuals with EDS access the equipment they need for daily living.

These tools and support networks are critical in assisting EDS patients and their families in better understanding the illness, obtaining effective care, and obtaining emotional support. Individuals with EDS should investigate and use these services to improve their general well-being and quality of life.

Chapter 5: Research, Future Directions, and Advocacy

The Current Areas of Research In Eds

Ehlers-Danlos Syndrome (EDS) is a developing field of study, and continuing research strives to increase our understanding of the disorder, its underlying causes, and prospective therapies. Some of the current research areas in EDS include:

1. Genetic Research:

- Genetic studies are being conducted to investigate the various genetic mutations associated with EDS subtypes. Researchers are discovering new genes and mutations that shed light on the genetic basis of the disease.

2. Connective Tissue Biology:

- It is critical to conduct research on the biology of connective tissues. Researchers are investigating how changes in collagen and other connective tissue components contribute to EDS symptoms.

3. Diagnostic Criteria and categorization:

- Researchers are attempting to improve EDS diagnostic criteria and create a more reliable categorization system that includes all EDS subtypes.

4. Pain Management:

- EDS patients frequently experience chronic pain. Studies are being conducted to develop effective pain management strategies, which may include medications, physical therapy, and alternative therapies.

5. Cardiac and Vascular Aspects:

- Research is being conducted to investigate the cardiac and vascular implications of EDS, particularly in the vascular subtype. It is critical for patient care to understand the cardiovascular risks associated with EDS.

6. Orthopedic and Surgical Interventions:

- Orthopedic research seeks surgical and non-surgical methods to stabilize joints and minimize the incidence of dislocations.

Comorbid Conditions:

- EDS is frequently accompanied by comorbid diseases such as dysautonomia, gastrointestinal problems, and mast cell activation syndrome. Researchers are examining the links between EDS and various disorders.

8. Quality of Life and Psychosocial Elements:

- Studies are looking at the psychosocial elements of living with EDS, including mental health issues, coping techniques, and quality of life. This research can assist in enhancing support for patients.

9. Rare Illness Collaboration:

- Collaboration with other rare illness groups is expanding since EDS shares parallels with other connective tissue disorders. Researchers are learning from these relationships to increase their understanding of EDS.

10. Medications and Treatment techniques:

- Research is studying prospective medications and treatment techniques, including the development of pharmaceuticals targeting particular parts of EDS pathogenesis.

11. **Patient-Driven Research:**

- Patient advocacy and patient-driven research efforts are playing an increasingly major role in EDS research. Patients are helping to research by sharing their experiences and data.

12. **Advocacy and Awareness:**

- Advocacy and awareness efforts are crucial in boosting the profile of EDS and fighting for improved research funding and assistance.

As our knowledge of EDS grows, these study areas show promise for improving the diagnosis, care, and overall quality of life for those with EDS. It is crucial for researchers, healthcare providers, and patient advocates to continue working together to promote advancement in the area and eventually provide better treatment for individuals living with EDS.

Ways Patients, Caregivers, and Healthcare Professionals Can Help Promote EDS Research and Awareness

A collaborative effort including patients, caregivers, and healthcare professionals is required to advance Ehlers-Danlos Syndrome (EDS) research and awareness. Below are some ways that each group may help to improve understanding and raise awareness about EDS:

1. Patients:

- **Participate in Research:** Think about taking part in EDS-related research studies and clinical trials. Your participation can assist researchers in gathering crucial data to further understand the illness.

- **Share Personal Experiences:** Sharing your own EDS journey and experiences might help to improve awareness and decrease stigma. It may also make other sufferers feel less solitary, encouraging them to seek care and a diagnosis.

- **Advocate for EDS:** Become an EDS champion by contacting local and national lawmakers, healthcare organizations, and rare illness advocacy groups. Advocate for more funding for EDS research and improved healthcare access.

- **Join Support Groups:** Find EDS support groups in your area as well as online. These organizations provide a forum for people with EDS to share knowledge, experiences, and emotional support with others who understand the difficulties they face.

2. Caregivers:

- **Educate Yourself:** Caregivers may play an important part in educating themselves about EDS. Understanding the illness and its challenges can allow you to better assist and advocate for your EDS-affected loved one.

- **Accompany Your Loved One to Medical Appointments:** Accompany your loved one to medical appointments and be an active participant in their treatment. Take notes, ask questions, and make sure your loved one's needs are met.

- **Raise Awareness:** Inform your social network, community, and healthcare professionals about EDS. Caregivers may assist in guaranteeing that EDS is identified and understood by a larger audience by promoting awareness.

3. Healthcare Providers:

- **Stay informed:** Healthcare practitioners should remain up to speed on the newest EDS research and clinical guidelines. Understanding the illness and how to treat it is critical for optimal care.

- **Refer to Specialists:** Refer EDS patients to specialists who are knowledgeable about the disease, such as rheumatologists, geneticists, or physical therapists, if needed. Develop thorough treatment strategies in collaboration with these professionals.

- **Patient Advocacy:** Advocate on behalf of your EDS patients to ensure they receive timely and adequate care. Help them navigate the healthcare system and obtain essential assistance.

- **Participate in Research:** Healthcare workers can actively participate in EDS research, clinical studies, and educational efforts if possible. The exchange of clinical knowledge and data can help to increase our understanding and management of EDS.

4. All Stakeholders:

- **Assist Advocacy Efforts:** Assist or participate in advocacy groups and projects that focus on EDS. These organizations are vital in raising awareness, sponsoring research, and pushing for legislative changes that will help EDS patients.

- **Educate the Public:** Disseminate EDS information and resources to the general public in order to raise awareness and comprehension of the illness. This can assist in shortening the time it takes to diagnose someone and enhance support for people who are impacted.

- **Encourage Early Diagnosis:** Encourage healthcare practitioners to explore EDS in individuals exhibiting similar symptoms and to refer them to experts for examination. An earlier diagnosis may result in better outcomes.

Patients, caregivers, and healthcare professionals may all work together to advance EDS research, promote awareness, and enhance the lives of those living with the illness. We can only increase our understanding of EDS and provide better support and care for people afflicted if we all work together.

The Future of Eds Therapy and Management

The future of Ehlers-Danlos Syndrome (EDS) therapy and management offers great potential for enhancing the quality of life for those suffering from the disorder. While there is no cure for EDS, continued research and improvements in medical technology are leading to improved therapy and management options. Below are some important developments for EDS on the horizon:

1. Tailored treatment strategies:

- As our understanding of EDS subtypes and individual variability grows, tailored treatment strategies become more practical. These programs will be adapted to the individual EDS subtype and symptom profile of each patient.

2. Genetic Therapies:

- There is continuing research into the genetic basis of EDS. Gene-based treatments may provide tailored therapy options for some EDS subtypes in the future. Gene therapy, while still in the experimental stage, provides promise for treating the underlying genetic mutations.

3. Pain Management Advancements:

- Pain management research for EDS is leading to more effective techniques for treating chronic pain. Pain medicines, physical therapy approaches, and alternative therapies are intended to enhance EDS patients' quality of life.

4. Joint Stabilization Techniques:

- Orthopedic and surgical therapies are advancing, with an emphasis on enhancing joint stability and lowering the likelihood of dislocations. EDS sufferers will benefit from advancements in surgical procedures and non-invasive joint stabilizing approaches.

5. Awareness and Education:

- As knowledge of EDS grows, healthcare practitioners will become more competent at recognizing the disease. Early detection is critical for improved care and the avoidance of problems.

6. Supportive Communities:

- The number of online and in-person support networks for EDS sufferers is growing. These communities offer useful information, emotional support, and a forum for knowledge sharing.

7. Rare Disease Collaboration:

- It is envisaged that collaboration between rare illness communities, including EDS, will expand.

Researchers will learn from the similarities and differences in various illnesses, which might lead to insights and therapies that are applicable to numerous ailments.

8. Advocacy and Funding:

- In the future further advocacy activities as well as greater funding for EDS research. These measures will fuel research and guarantee that EDS gets the attention it deserves.

9. Telemedicine and Remote Care:

- Telemedicine and remote healthcare services are anticipated to play an important role in EDS management, particularly for patients with restricted mobility or access to specialized EDS clinics.

10. Patient-Driven Research:

- Patient-driven research and clinical study participation are projected to become increasingly widespread. Patients can actively contribute to our understanding of EDS and play an important role in directing research.

While these advancements provide promise for improved EDS care, it is crucial to realize that improvement may be slow. EDS is still a complicated and multidimensional disorder, and progress will be built on a foundation of study and collaboration. Individuals with EDS, healthcare professionals, and advocacy groups will all play critical roles in promoting future treatment and management options.

Organizations and Advocacy Groups That Offer Eds Support

Several organizations and advocacy groups exist to support, raise awareness, and advocate for people with Ehlers-Danlos Syndrome (EDS). The following are some significant EDS organizations and advocacy groups:

1. **The Ehlers-Danlos Society:** The Ehlers-Danlos Society is a global organization dedicated to furthering EDS research, offering educational materials, and assisting people living with EDS. They host international conferences, support

research, and provide patients and healthcare professionals with a variety of tools.

2. **Ehlers-Danlos Support UK:** This UK-based nonprofit provides assistance, information, and advocacy to people with EDS and their families. They offer skilled medical advice as well as support groups.

3. **EDS Awareness:** EDS Awareness is a non-profit organization that works to raise awareness about EDS and associated disorders. They offer materials and organize support groups.

4. **The Hypermobility Disorders Association (HMSA):** The HMSA is a UK-based organization that assists people suffering from hypermobility disorders such as EDS. They provide knowledge, advocacy, and assistance.

5. **The Zebra Network:** This group unites people with uncommon diseases, such as EDS, and offers support and information. They also provide a forum for people to share their tales.

6. **EDS Today:** EDS Today is an online community committed to raising awareness, offering support, and sharing information on EDS and associated illnesses.

7. **The Marfan Foundation:** The Marfan Foundation generally focuses on Marfan syndrome, but it also provides vital materials and assistance to those with EDS because the diseases are comparable.

8. **The Rare Diseases Clinical Research Network (RDCRN):** RDCRN is a network of research consortia centered in the United States committed to promoting research on rare diseases such as EDS. Their findings might lead to a better understanding of EDS and better treatment options.

9. **National Organization for Rare Disorders (NORD):** NORD is a non-profit organization established in the United States that promotes people suffering from rare diseases. They provide patient aid services, as well as information and resources.

10. **Global Genes:** Global Genes is a global rare illness advocacy group that raises awareness, fosters collaboration, and provides support to people living with rare diseases such as EDS.

These organizations and advocacy groups are critical in connecting people with EDS, giving support and information, and lobbying for better treatment and research funding. Depending on where you live, you may be able to identify local or regional groups that provide further support and services to people with EDS and their families.

CONCLUSION

The goal of this book was to shed light on the complicated and sometimes misunderstood realm of Ehlers-Danlos Syndrome (EDS). We've looked at the basics of EDS, its numerous kinds, and the diagnosis procedure, as well as how it impacts people physically, emotionally, and intellectually. We've presented a holistic picture of EDS and how to navigate life with this illness through conversations on symptom management and the significance of emotional well-being.

We've talked about the newest research, the future of EDS care, and the power of activism, highlighting the necessity of cooperation and common knowledge in the EDS community.

As we weave these threads together, keep in mind that EDS is more than simply a medical illness; it affects the lives of many people and their families. While it poses unique problems, it also demonstrates human perseverance and tenacity. It serves as a reminder that we can adapt, grow, and prosper in the face of hardship.

We'd want to leave you with this thought: EDS isn't a restriction; it's an opportunity for progress and a cry for increased knowledge and support. Each individual with EDS has a unique story to share, and we want you to listen to them, learn from them, and join the network that makes life with EDS not just bearable, but also tremendously enjoyable.

May this book serve as a beacon of knowledge and empathy, helping to create a society in which EDS is not only recognized but also accepted with compassion and inclusion. Thank you for joining us on this trip, which we hope will encourage you to continue exploring the rich tapestry of human experiences.